Selected Journals of Successful Hospice Palliative Care

from the 16th International Congress on
Care of the Terminally Ill

Selected Journals of Successful Hospice Palliative Care

from the 16th International Congress on
Care of the Terminally Ill
September 26-29, 2006 Montreal, Canada

Harry van Bommel, Editor

Legacies: Family and Community Resources

ISBN 1-55307-032-1

Library and Archives Canada Cataloguing in Publication
Selected journals of successful hospice palliative care:
16th International Congress on Care of the Terminally Ill,
September 26-29, 2006, Montreal, Canada / Harry van Bommel, editor.
Includes bibliographical references and index.
ISBN 1-55307-032-1
1. Palliative treatment. 2. Hospice care. 3. Terminal care.
4. Terminally ill. I. Van Bommel, Harry II. International Congress
on Care of the Terminally Ill (16th : 2006 : Montréal, Québec)
R726.8.S45 2006 362.17'5 C2006-905853-9

Legacies: Family and Community Resources
11 Miniot Circle, Scarborough Ontario M1K 2K1 Canada
Telephone 416.264.4665 Fax 800.684.7280
On the web at http://www.legacies.ca

Produced in association with the
Media Futures Institute

Table of Contents

This book is presented in alphabetical order by author's name.

Acknowledgements / 7
Introduction / 9

Adams, Lucie: **Measuring Time in Hours** / 11
Michéle Chaban: **Sam Federman – A Song Can Save Lives** / 15
Corbier, Melanie: **Oh No! Am I Still Here?** / 21
Cottle, Margaret: **We Can All Do Small Things with Love** / 25
Fillmore, Cathleen: **Implications of Mortality** / 27
Hartee, Colin: **The Difference Between Pain and Suffering** / 30
Holland, Joyce: **AFGOS** / 32
Holtzer, Andrea: **What it Means to 'Be There'** / 33
LaRocque, Elizabeth: **Hospice-Palliative Care IS The Weaned Child on the Lap** / 36
Leece, Suzanne: **Joanna's Story** / 38
MacDonald, Colleen: **Warm Hands** / 40
Macková, Marie: **Guardian Angel** / 43
Mount, Balfour: **The Ten Commandments of Healing** / 45
Murray, Mary: **A Job Where Everybody Dies** / 50
Paddon, Elizabeth: **Leave with a Grace** / 54
Ruiter, Nick: **A Hospice Client Encounter** / 56
Rutenberg, Mona: **Handcasting: Holding onto a Legacy** / 57
Schleinich, Mary Anne: **Reconnecting to Her Whole** / 59
Smith, Ian R.: **Ruth: An Interfaith Encounter** / 61
Stark, Janet: **Coming Home** / 64
Towers, Anna: **Touch Their Hand Gently** / 67
van Bommel, Harry: **Let's Go for a Walk** / 68

Index / 72

Dedication

This book is dedicated in memory of **Dame Cicely Saunders**, founder of the modern hospice palliative care movement. Her death last year reminded so many of us that the movement begins and ends with "watch with me." Watch with me to meet the physical, spiritual, emotional and information needs of people nearing the end of their lives as well as the needs of their families, and professional and volunteer care providers. Her presence is sadly missed.

In honor of **Balfour Mount,** founder and ongoing inspiration of the *International Congress on Care of the Terminally Ill* and a pioneer of the hospice palliative care movement in Canada and internationally. He has helped, encouraged and supported countless individuals and organizations to develop programs and services that meet the needs of patients and their families to live life fully. His continuing gift of teaching others how to care for patients, families and professional and volunteer care providers leaves a lasting legacy.

Acknowledgements

The organizing committee of the *16th International Congress on Care of the Terminally Ill* made it possible, through their organizers, **April Donahue** and **Robert O'Donoughue**, to collect these stories from Congress participants. Without their efforts, this book would not have been possible.

The Congress Executive Committee was:

Anna Towers, Congress Chair and Director, Palliative Care Division, Department of Oncology and Medicine, McGill University, Montreal.

Robin Cohen, SMBD Jewish General Hospital, Director of Research, Palliative Care Division, Departments of Oncology and Medicine, McGill University, Montreal.

Kappy Flanders, Co-Chair, Council on Palliative Care, Montreal.

Bernard Lapointe, Director of Palliative Care, SMBD Jewish General Hospital, Montreal.

The Congress Programme Committee was:

Nathalie Aubin, Montreal General Hospital, (McGill University Health Centre), Montreal.

Manny Borod, McGill University Health Centre, Montreal.

Martin Chasen, Royal Victoria Hospital, (McGill University Health Centre), Montreal

Linda Crelinsten, McGill University, Montreal.

Johanne de Montigny, Montreal General Hospital, (McGill University Health Centre), Montreal.

Justine Farley, St. Mary's Hospital, Montreal.

Krista Lawlor, McGill University Health Centre, Montreal.

Diane Lebeau, McGill University Health Centre, Montreal.

Stephen Liben, The Montreal Children's Hospital, (McGill University Health Centre), Montreal.

Kelli Stajduhar, University of Victoria, Victoria (BC).

Golda Tradounsky, Mount Sinai Hospital Centre, Montreal.

Raymond Viola, Kingston General Hospital, Queen's University, Kingston (ON).

The Congress Programme Advisors were:
Balfour M. Mount, Emeritus Professor of Medicine, McGill University
Neil MacDonald, Professor, McGill University.
William Lawlor, Professor (retired), McGill University.

Several other people deserve special mention for their timely help:
Robert Macdonald designed this book for publication and has put in on our web site (http://www.legacies.ca) to share with all Congress participants and anyone interested in successful hospice palliative care around the world. He worked quickly and effectively to bring this information to a global audience within two weeks of the Congress's meetings. Thank you so much Robert.

All of the **O'Donoughue & Associates Event Management Ltd.** staff and volunteers were wonderfully helpful and encouraging. Specific thanks to:

Gracia Jalea for ensuring that copies of the requests to delegates to share their stories got into every delegate's package with extra copies available in the Internet Café at the conference.

Frank Salvatori for allowing me time on his Internet account to work on this book while also generously providing excellent web site design ideas so we can reach an even wider audience.

Lastly my sincere appreciation to **Gwen Klees** and **Robert Croteau** for their hospitality while I was in Montreal and **Janet**, **Bram** and **Joanna** for encouraging me to take the six days away from our family to work on this project.

Introduction

First an apology – the stories in this book were collected during 4 days of the 16th International Congress on Care of the Terminally Ill in Montreal, Canada. The short time frame may well lead to a few grammatical and typing errors that were not caught in the editing and proofreading process. I apologize to the writers of this book for any unintentional errors. Please send me any corrections for a revised edition that will be updated and posted on our web page http://www.legacies.ca.

The format of the book has been purposely kept very simple for easy use by delegates of the conference to use the material in their own word-processing or publishing software. The stories are alphabetical, by author's name and the index includes both authors' names and topic headings.

The stories in this book look at the physical, emotional, spiritual and information aspects of care; views by professionals about their work; personal stories by spouses, parents, children and siblings; and even some philosophical musings.

You are encouraged to read the stories and use them in your work. For example, you might use some of the stories in your newsletters, annual reports, other publications, teachings, or to help colleagues or clients understand a specific point about the hospice palliative care philosophy of care.

You are further encouraged to keep on writing your stories and sharing them with others. Through stories we come alive in our work and in our own perspective of the importance of hospice palliative care. Using the Internet and other means, we can share our stories with colleagues, quickly all over the world.

NB: Unless otherwise stated, the names of people in the following stories have been changed to protect their privacy and that of their families and care providers.

Leo Tolstoy wrote that every time we write we should leave "a bit of our blood in the inkpot." The stories in this book do exactly that. The stories are thoughtful, personal and a great testament to the importance of human relationships in all their many forms. I am grateful to the writers for sharing their stories with all of us.

What You Must Do to Use the Stories in Your Work

This material was gathered at and for the16th International Congress on Care of the Terminally Ill, September 26-29, 2006 in Montreal, Canada. Everyone who has participated in the project has ensured that their stories are free of error and respect the confidentiality of the people involved as necessary. They retain copyright for their own stories and accept responsibility for what is recorded. Conference participants, and other interested parties, are free to copy whatever material they feel would be helpful in promoting excellence in care. Other than the publisher, Legacies Inc., they cannot sell the book. If they wish to edit or revise any story, they must contact the storyteller directly for permission. If they include this material in other published formats (e.g. as part of a book), they must acknowledge its source. Anyone who uses this material is asked to inform the original author and the publisher, Legacies Inc., in writing and to send a sample of how the material was used to each. The correct citation for reproducing any part of this book is:

Author's last name, first name or initials. (September 2006). "Title" in *Selected Journals of Successful Hospice Palliative Care from the 16th International Congress on Care of the Terminally Ill, September 26-29, 2006 in Montreal, Canada*. Toronto: Legacies Inc.

Lucie Adams

Measuring Time in Hours

The first time we saw Monique, she'd just been told she had advanced cancer. She was also going to go to Oncology for some chemo, possibly, but she came to us, at the Palliative Care outpatient clinic, sent by the Palliative Care physician who saw her at Lung Clinic, that day.

It was late afternoon, April, rainy, and I needed to complete my paperwork, lock up the clinic, pick up my husband and go home. It had been a long day.

But then, Monique walked in, with her tardive diagnosis, alone, panting, pushing back her waist-length black hair, and I invited her to sit. She chose a straight chair, the most uncomfortable one, like she planned not to stay long.

Whatever time she actually spent with me went by so fast! A workaholic attorney in her early forties, Monique uttered nothing that didn't matter. Long into her assessment, she told me she was about to marry for the first time, so I stood up, pulled my chair closer, and congratulated her heartily, knowing full well that whomever she was marrying would soon be widowed...

She stayed breathless throughout that first visit, but paid it no mind – she allowed this difficulty in breathing very little space. She was so articulate. She spoke as if she were writing the final draft of an essay. I found her a joy to listen to. I forgot to take notes.

At some point in an article on Palliative Care, I'd read that you have to love the patients fast. Well, I wanted to love Monique even faster, because I wouldn't have minded hearing more of her story at that first meeting. To think I just wanted to go home after my clinic! To think I could have not met Monique! To think, really, that nobody would have made my day if it hadn't been for her...

Monique was, if nothing else, fully determined to survive her 3-month prognosis. She was going to prove to everyone that miracles do happen.

She began chemo, and, alongside that, we were managing her pain. Her cancer was spreading; her response to chemo was poor, and the disease continued to ravage her. Interestingly, before starting chemo, Monique had her beautiful tresses cut off so she could donate the hair to make a wig. But the wig wouldn't be for her. It would be for a cancer patient undergoing chemo! As if she, herself, wasn't that cancer patient! As if she, herself, would be completely cured, and her own hair would grow back...

How I loved her stoicism, and her business-like lack of drama! How I admired her courage! How I felt awe at her humble, selfless generosity!

When I met her boyfriend in May, a man younger than herself, I said very little to him, and figured that Monique may have guessed at my disapproval of him. These things never get spoken, but they do get said, somehow, when you're "loving them fast"...He was needy, and she was dying. This looked, if anything, like a most incompatible union. My heart sank for her. But never mind. She had to live this bit of life she had left. She had to live it her way.

Monique's latest scan showed brain metastasis, but this news anchored her in becoming even more relentless with her plan to live. With her parents deceased, and her sister not really that close, she held on, fiercely, to her independence and autonomy. Never did she talk about the law practice that had been her consummate passion for so many years....What she did talk about was the new house she'd bought in the country, and how much she would enjoy relaxing in the hot tub she'd ordered.

She was becoming weaker, more tired, more drowsy. Also, there was more pain, but talk about her symptoms was terse, cursory, almost dismissive.

Her boyfriend left her. She'd made all her arrangements, and then, the June wedding never happened. The break-up started over a silly argument about something she'd lost, or temporarily misplaced, having put it at the back of a drawer. She cried. I touched her. She felt warm, maybe even feverish, but her temperature was of no concern, compared to her broken heart.

At the end of June, Monique moved in with her sister, brother-in-law and young children. Her sister, a primary school teacher, knew nothing about the care Monique needed, wished Monique would agree to be admitted to a facility, but didn't have the heart to tell her this....It was as if she wanted me to inject her, or infuse her, with some hope for their whole family; as if hope were a commodity that could be shared among all of them, equally. As if hope brought the same satisfaction a chocolate fix might. As if it would all go away, this business. As if Monique were not going to die. As if life would go back to before Monique got sick....

But there was no magic solution. At the clinic, we'd seen Monique maybe 8 times total, and with each visit, the deterioration in her condition was markedly noticeable. She was changing fast. Dying. And she wanted to be at home, or at her sister's home, which now had become hers because she could no longer care for herself, couldn't feed, wash, toilet herself, had blurred vision, and was spending all of her days and nights in bed, diapered, just trying to breathe. She was getting oxygen at home. She had a visit scheduled for mid-July with us.

Right after the Canada Day holiday, I got a call from the community health clinic nurse who'd gone to the home. Monique couldn't swallow anymore, and was receiving her medication subcutaneously, through a butterfly needle, which her sister had been taught to use. Monique was spending her time in a state of confusion and disorientation, but she was not agitated. She was calm, and awoke for briefer and briefer periods of time...I asked to speak to Monique, if she was awake, and if that was okay, and her sister put me on. In her weak, feeble whisper, she said her hello to me and announced that she was in bed. What a joy it was to have her remember me through the murky terrain her once-sharp mind had become! I had the chance to thank her for being her. I knew her for the last three months of her life, and our therapeutic relationship had lasted hours, the hours of her clinic visits.

Monique died a few days after that, as she'd lived, passionately attached to that which was important, at the moment it was important. She died with her family close by. She died having made friends with her sister's tears.

I worried about Monique's sister and was getting ready to arrange for bereavement follow-up when a bouquet of flowers arrived at the clinic, thanking us for everything we did for Monique, and for their whole family. I knew, then, that everything was going to be all right.

It was when the letter of condolence to Monique's sister was brought to me to sign, that my eyes welled up and spilled over, but just for a terse, cursory moment....

Lucie Adams, RN, BA
McGill University Health Center, Palliative Care
4 Yuile Street, Kirkland, QC H9H 5K6 CANADA
514.693.0542, misslu16@yahoo.com

Michéle Chaban

Sam Federman – A Song Can Save Lives

I had been working on a cancer floor for some years when I met Sam (his real name used with permission). Our team had come to identify those who had a potential history of harm and so as a matter of course, if one of the team felt this might be an issue, an automatic referral was made to social work.

When I first set eyes on Sam he was lying in bed, sheets pulled up to his neck. His nose hung over the fold of the sheets. It seemed like a pose that accompanied sheer fear. His wife sat beside him in his room. I introduced myself. Only the twinkling of Sam's eyes, the wrinkling and crinkling of his face denoted a smile .

When I introduced myself, the sheets came down and then I saw Sam Federman's glorious face shining like a rising sun. He emulated life and joy. I thought this could hardly be a man who had been through the kind of harm and hurt that so often accompanies the survivorship of war and incarceration. Sam listened to my description of our team and our service as I asked if there was anything I might do to help him. He was most appreciative of my time and my efforts. He thanked me profusely. On the day of surgery his two fine sons and his mother paced the hall, waiting for him. When he arrived they hovered protectively. This intensity seemed familiar, reflective of the others who had not only come to the floor for surgery but who had a history of having been in concentration camps.

I approached one of his sons. As I did so he thanked me for all that I had done. I was not quite sure I had done anything. I said "please think nothing of it, it is how we work around here as a team". He then said his "father had been terrified of coming in for surgery but that there had been an extra something in everyone he had met that made him feel he was not only safe but that his fear was deeply understood". I then took the opportunity to ask Sam's son "where was your father during the war"?

His son looked deeply into me, one of those searching looks that animals send out as they sniff the air and ask if they might trust what they sense as your being. He then said "Aushwitz". I looked to the floor and said "I see, we thought that might be the case and that was why we were so protective". He then asked "how we knew" ? I said "we didn't , we just have seen a lot of holocaust survivors on the floor coming in with illness, we don't know if it was the conditions in the camps, what they ate, or the starvation they endured, but now they have problems with their gastro-intestinal system."

Later, I would talk to Sam about how we might have made it easier for him and his family to undergo surgery. He assured me that the team had accomplished its goal. It seemed to me if we had done well, he never should have had the sheets all the way up to his nose in the first five minutes of being on our floor. Then again, if I had endured what Sam had endured, I might never have made it to the floor.

Over the coarse of time Sam told me his story. Sam was a young boy when he was taken to the camps with his family. His father and uncle protected him as much as they could. In the camps the stronger men were used to bury bodies. Each night, the men were put onto the back of a truck and taken to a hidden part of the forest where they were instructed to unload and bury the bodies that had died that day. The men knew that young Sam's survivorship depended on his helping them do this gruesome task. So each night his father and his uncle as well as the men around them, helped Sam seem more productive than he was in reality.

One night, the Nazis decided that some of the men were not carrying their own weight and so they buried them alive. Sam's father was one of them.

Later that night some of the prisoners stole back to see if any of those buried alive could be saved. Before he died , Sam's father asked the men of the camp to care for his son as if he was their own. They did.

Winter set in and burying became more difficult. On Christmas eve, the commandant and some of his men came to the barracks. They had been drinking.

It was a high and holy day and they were away from their families. They were sad and sentimental, lonely and angry to be separated from those they loved.

They came to take their feelings out on others. They came to shoot a few men for the sport of it.

One of the officers ordered that everyone get out of bed for an inspection. The prisoners lined up, fearful of what was next. The officers inspected the prisoners eyeing the ones that might be the recipients of their bullets. Sam was beside himself. His father had always taught him that something could be done when a bad situation was getting worse. Sam stepped forward out of the line of men. The older men around him gasped and reached for him, but the officers pushed them back. Sam stood before the commandant. The commandant looked down on him. Sam began to sing the only Christmas carol he knew from his home town. Sam sang with all the power and soul his lungs could muster.

He invested each word with joy and hope and love. This little Jewish boy sang with the spirit of Christmas, filling the barracks.

The commandant's eyes filled with tears. The other officers shifted about, with similar discomfort for what had just taken place. The commandant asked for the boy's name. Sam stepped closer and looking down at the floor he then quietly stated his name. The commandant said "Sam

Federman, tonight your song has saved lives". The commandant turned and left the barracks, his men were ordered to follow.

Sam survived the camps although most of his family did not. When I met him, I think he was well into his 70's. He had married and had two sons. In his retirement, Sam would visit nursing homes and sing to those who now spent their life in institutional care. I asked why he did that. He said " a song can save a life".

I was so impressed with the life that Sam Federman lived and the spirit with which he embraced life that I thought something should be done to honor his humanitarianism. I spoke to the Rabbi at our hospital about my thoughts. I wanted Sam's story to go down in history. I wanted his story to be told.

After the war and after some time had come to pass, there had been an attempt to document the atrocities of the camp survivors. Sam told me that he had told his story to a documentarian. I asked if I might see it. Sam gave me a copy of the interview. It was a sad reminder of the suffering that Sam had endured. It was an even sadder reminder of our witnessing to his suffering. The interviewer sat passively and unmoved as Sam told his story, as Sam wept and wailed over his losses. Perhaps in those days, the ideas was to capture the story and storyteller and not allow the narrator to intrude upon the story. Yet once again, humanity stood by and watched as Sam suffered alone. I did not want this to be the last testament to Sam's life.

I had heard rumors about Steven Speilberg's "righteous man" award. I did not know more about it than its name but surely Sam Federman was a righteous man. The money from Schindlers List was being used to support the award. I set out to find out more about it. In the process of doing so, others started to make inquiries. In the end, I believe it was one of Sam's sons who made the arrangements.

One day, Steven Speilberg's crew arrived at Sam Federman's house. They set up their lights and cameras and they asked that Sam tell his story once again. This time, no witness remained unmoved. Sam told the story of how a song saves a life. Sam told the story about how it sometimes only takes one person to save many. Sam told the story about how even the most wicked of hearts can be turned if you dare to know them for their broken hearted ways rather than their wickedness, if you dare to offer them what their heart most seeks. At the end of his story, Sam called his sons to him. Both walk onto the set, standing behind their father. The meaning was clear.

Sam's father, his uncle, and the men that lived in the barracks had a legacy of helping each other, helping to remind others what was right and wrong even amidst such evil. Sam had survived because of the help of strangers.

Sam in turn had helped strangers to survive then and now, with his song. Sam had lived and given birth to another generation . The legacy of love and protectionism that had been taught to him by his father and his uncle was clearly passed onto his sons. It was evident at the time of Sam's surgery and evident in the film as his sons stood longingly and protectively near their father.

Sam and I would have many conversations as he came and went from the hospital over the years. A few weeks before Sam died of his cancer he sent me a copy of the film made by Steven Speilberg's organization and gave me permission to use his story to teach. He also had a tree planted in Israel in my name. I felt this was a tremendous honor that one such as Sam should pay tribute to me. I have had many occasions to tell Sam's story when I am faced with people's sense of despair around world events or the unfairness of a death in a family. I always conclude the story by saying "sometimes it only takes one person's song to change the world". Now that Sam can no longer sing, I would say "sometimes it only takes Sam's story to change a heart".

Chaban, Michéle. (September 2006). "Sam Federman – A Song Can Save Lives" in *Selected Journals of Successful Hospice Palliative Care from the 16th International Congress on Care of the Terminally Ill, September 26-29, 2006 in Montreal, Canada*. Toronto: Legacies Inc.

Michéle Chaban, MSW, RSW, DPhil
PhD Supervisor, University of Wales
Post Graduate Supervisor, University of Toronto, School of Social Work
Post Grad at Wilfred Laurier University
International Lecturer and Speaker
CANADA
416.533.1976, michele.chaban@utoronto.ca

Melanie Corbier

Oh No! Am I Still Here?

My Mom. Eighty years old, pack-a-day smoker for 60 years, an avid gardener, mother of three, grandmother of 12. She was living alone (Dad had died five years previously) content with her dog as best friend, in a small community where all the shopkeepers knew their customers and Mom was a well-known figure on her daily walk to the Post Office.

When she was diagnosed with cancer of the lung, her first reaction was "Oh, good. I won't stroke and lie in a bed for 10 years," (her worst fear).

She decided on no treatment. "I'm 80 years old, had a good life, brought this on myself by smoking, and I have to die of something. Cancer of the lung is what it will be."

She had always regarded dying and a new life as the ultimate adventure, and was sure she would be joining Dad and others who had gone before. Having decided on no treatment, her next decision was to be open about her future with her friends, family and community. This openness brought the whole community into an unofficial support group over the next two years, as she visibly declined in health.

She also declared she had not time for this problem right now. She had contracted with her teenage grandson to re-build a large garden for the following June. It was to be all blooming in pink for a wedding and there was no time to lose.

I decided to start homecare services, starting with a homemaker, as I was spending quite a lot of time doing chores for Mom. We got a wonderful, tough, big-hearted woman, whose previous job was bartending in a local hotel! She wasn't very experienced as a homemaker but she was very willing and quick to learn. She was extremely funny with a wicked wit. She stayed 'til Mom died and we leaned on her in countless ways.

During that summer Mom worked on this huge garden project with her grandson being the muscles. As she got weaker over the summer, she did more supervising than work, but she never missed a day, until the snow came in late November.

Winter came and went. Except for fatigue (daily rests after lunch) she remained quite well. As soon as the frost was out of the ground, she and her helper swung into full gear, as they struggled to get this garden blooming for June.

Fortunately, it was an early spring. All the fall plantings came alive. The bulbs came up, the shrubs came into flower and the perennials actually bloomed on time. It was a huge success and brought a great deal of attention and admiration for the gardener and her helper. It was a crowning achievement!

For the rest of the summer she and her grandson worked on her own garden which had been neglected for most of the year. She felt fine, just tired and needing to rest after lunch, which she resented. She still walked to town several days a week. Winter arrived and she felt the cold badly. Her community cared well for her. When she was suddenly overcome with weakness in the Post Office, a kind man upended the garbage bin and sat her down until it passed. The variety store owner took one look at her another and said, "Mrs. C., are you alright?" She asked the next customer who came through the door to drive her home, which he willingly did. She was in good hands at all times.

Unbelievably, she made it to another spring. She was in a state of bliss to see her beloved flowers "one more time." Every bulb that came up, every flower that opened was a fresh miracle to her. That summer she really was obviously failing. Her color was gray, her weight dropped and her appetite was poor. She sat outside, unable to work but content.

My sister arrived during this summer to stay until Mom died. This solved the problem of Mom alone at night. She was getting pretty shaky on her feet. My sister and Mom created a book, with one page for each room of the small house. On each page was listed the contents of the room with a place where she could indicate who was to receive each item. She spent many happy hours bequeathing her many beautiful treasures to her loved ones.

As the summer drew to a close, many old friends and family came to see her and to say goodbye. They were a little unsettled by her openly talking and waiting "to go." She was getting impatient to see her loved ones and to see what the next life was all about. She remained symptom free, (continued to smoke, of course) only expressing a fear of pain. She never had any pain, nor any shortness of breath. As she became more impatient to die, we found ourselves saying things like, "Don't worry Mom. I'm sure you'll be dying soon," and "Just be patient, the end is in sight." This felt a little strange but we were definitely all walking together. She wanted to go on, so we were the cheering section. We laughed ourselves silly over all sorts of family jokes, daily events, decreasing activity levels; you name it.

Three weeks before her death, there was a marked change. She ate less, moved less, spent more time lying down. Any activity exhausted her. Her sense of humor sharpened and our homemaker was in her element. We were all a great team.

Two weeks before her death, a very friend 15 years her junior, died in a freak car accident. When we told her the news, she was quiet for a moment. Then she said, "She got there before I did," in wondering tones.

The last week of her life she was down to skin and bones and increasingly weak. She found her bed more and more comfortable so there she spent most of her time. I had also moved into her house and we set up a rooster of friends who sat the night shift for us. Mom was awake often at night and although she was still pain free, she was restless and needed to drink. Several times as I sat by her side, she would stop breathing and the hand I was holding would go cold, even a little bit blue. I would whisper, "It's okay to go Mom." Then she would take a big breath, open her eyes and sigh, "I thought I was going. Why can't I just get going?" She was really frustrated about being stuck here!

One morning, I was by her side as she awoke. She looked sleepily up in my face and said, "Oh no!" I said, "What's wrong Mom?" as she sounded very distressed. She said, "Am I still here?" I laughed and said, "You're still talking Mom so I guess you're still here." She resigned herself to living another day.

The last morning of her life she awoke but answered us from far away when we spoke to her. She drifted back into a sleep-like state breathing gently and peacefully. Then she just didn't take another breath. We held our collective breath not daring to believe she was finally on her way! The mood in the house was joy and triumph. We did it! Mom had died happily, peacefully, at home, with her family by her side.

Our favourite V.O.N. nurse walked through the door for her daily visit. We greeted her with laughter saying she was too late. Mom was gone! I remember feeling like we had all just won the race of our lives. Mom had finally made it! She was home!

Melanie Corbier
R.R. #2, Colborne, ON K0K 1S0 CANADA
905.335.3401

Margaret Cottle

We Can All Do Small Things with Love

The photos at her bedside record a family picnic: the children laughing and Susan and her husband Tom embracing—her long thick hair shining in the sunlight.

The picnic and the hair are now only a memory. Lying in her hospital bed with crumbling bones and a bald head, she glances at the photo and says quietly, "My hair was beautiful once..."

So many losses, but her deepest source of grief is leaving Tom and the children alone.

The members of their small church courageously share the difficult journey, faithfully expressing their love for the family in a many practical ways. One way, however, is particularly memorable.

Each of the four children, ages three to ten, has a special friend in different families at church. These families "adopt" one of Tom and Susan's children for at least a year after Susan's death. Soccer teams, piano lessons, birthday parties, trips to the park, school shopping, Scouts, swimming lessons, hair cuts, church, whatever the activities, Susan's children are included.

They live and sleep at home with their dad, but keep toys, clothes and pyjamas at their second "home" for "emergencies." This arrangement makes it easier for Tom to return to work,
frees up time for him to spend with the children at home and gives him space to grieve.

Before her death, Susan is profoundly comforted by her friends' commitment to her family. Thousands of small kindnesses follow.

The mother or father at the wheel of the car may consider transporting an extra child to soccer practice on a rainy afternoon insignificant. Mother Teresa knew better. She said, "We cannot all do great things, but we can all do small things with great love."

Margaret Cottle
4574 W 15th Ave., Vancouver, BC V6R 3B4 CANADA
604.222.0288, mmcottle@mac.com

Cathleen Fillmore

Implications of Mortality

It was twenty-five years ago, when my mother called from Florida in mid-day. I knew immediately something was up. We stumbled through the mandatory small talk as I waited for her real message.

And here it was. She'd been diagnosed with breast cancer. There was, as she knew there would be, a stunned silence at my end. My first thoughts, I admit, were of myself and the terrible loss I was now threatened with. Without warning, mortality had shoved his thick ugly tongue down my throat.

After pulling up some platitudes, I hung up and tried to compose myself.

I was raising two children so holding it together was important. But my life, my world, were now in a long-term spin cycle.

When colleagues asked about my mother, I said "She's doing well." I sounded calm as I restrained my feral self from acting out what I *really* felt like doing – screaming, smashing windows and throwing myself on the floor in utter despair.

How mature is that?

It gets even weirder. For several months, my concern for my mother's health was dominant in my mind and I wrote and phoned her faithfully. Then I'd skip a week or two. Things went back to normal and the ambivalence I often felt about my mother crept back. She really could be annoying!

My younger son and I went to visit my parents in Florida for a week. My mother seemed to be holding her own as I gratefully slipped into the soporific comfort of denial. She had years ahead of her. Sure.

On the last day of my visit, I was sitting on the patio and overheard her tell a friend what she would never say to me, "I had such a sharp pain in my chest today, the worst pain I've ever felt."

A dagger flew into my chest and stuck there for months.

Fast forward a few years....My parents were now living in their hometown of Moncton, New Brunswick. Florida had become a figment of my mother's imagination as she wistfully spoke of going back.

"No," said my father emphatically.

Slowly and with great resistance, she released her dreams one by one as her life now became the circumference of a full circle in her wheelchair.

One of the stories I grew up with is that my mother was rounding a corner one day with the sun hitting her eyes when a total stranger stopped her on the street as he blurted out in astonishment, "Madam, you have the bluest eyes I've ever seen."

And so she did. In the words of a much-quoted former beau, they were "like bluest water, seen through mists of rain."

Whenever she would lament the aging process, I'd remind her that as long as she had those eyes, she'd always be beautiful.

She no longer had those eyes. They reflected nothing back to me, neither bluest waters nor mists of rain. They'd become translucent, a Bermuda Triangle zone. I feared if I looked too deeply, I'd fall right in.

The last day of my week-long visit with my parents fell on April first. As I walked into my mother's bedroom, she smiled and said "I was wondering how to trick you."

Well might she wonder. Bed-ridden and mortally ill, what magical powers could she wield? What wand could that frail arm wave?

Yet in the end, she pulled off the ultimate trick. She evaporated into thin air.

Her absence created a crater that I have had to skirt around.

And yet, there's something else here, something a little more sinister.

When faced with my mother's mortality, my love for her became pure and selfless. During periods of her rallying, it was tempered with ambivalence.

Back and forth, picking petals off a daisy, "I love her, I love her not. I love her, I love her not." The ultimate petal, of course, the only *real* petal is "I love her."

It's exhausting to sustain intense love - kind of like a muscle we as a species haven't yet exercised enough. Grieving is a process of weaving mixed emotions in an entire pattern. Mortality is a gift, it helps us access unadulterated love.

When it's my turn to draw this incredibly rich journey to a close, I hope my children won't struggle so much with their feelings. I plan to give them permission to be as ambivalent as they please.

And it's true, I *can* be annoying.

Cathleen Fillmore
Journalist/author
President, Speakers' Gold
1463 Davenport Road, Suite 205, Toronto, ON M6H 2H6 CANADA
416.532.9886, cathleen.fillmore@rogers.com, www.speakersgold.com

Colin Hartree

The Difference Between Pain and Suffering

Albert was 75 years old when admitted to the hospice with mesothelioma and intractable chest wall pain. He was a retired hospital porter who had seen enough in his work to know that there was a prospect of a painful, difficult death.

On admission, he was cachectic, withdrawn, bitter and angry. He was difficult to engage in conversation and would answer questions as minimally as possible. He described no surviving family and no friends came to visit him.

It was my task as a junior doctor to attend to him daily and I usually put off seeing him as long as possible, so difficult and uncomfortable was it to engage with him and make any meaningful connection.

For his pain we tried increasing doses of opioids, alternative opioids, a variety of adjuvant analgesics including antidepressants but none of these pharmacological changes made any difference.

Cordotomy was not available locally but the pain clinic specialist visited and offered to insert a pleural catheter, something he could only do in three day's time.

I gradually learned that although he would talk about anything other than his illness, most of all, he preferred silent companionship. It was far from clear to me at the time that this had any therapeutic benefit.

Two days before the procedure, a distraught nurse called me to the bathroom where Albert was crying inconsolably. By now I knew better than to attempt any words and merely drew up a chair and sat beside him. Gradually the sobbing calmed and haltingly he began to talk. He explained that he knew he was dying and this in itself was not the cause of his distress. He went on to describe that thirty-five years ago he had had a big row with his son and they had not been in touch since. He was now fearful that he would die without ever seeing him again.

Fortunately, it was possible to contact his son who duly came to visit the next day. Following the visit, Albert was transformed. He complained of pain no more. It was possible to reduce his analgesic doses markedly and we cancelled the pleural catheter. He died peacefully six days after his son's visit.

I learned from Albert to distinguish pain and suffering, to realize that if medicines aren't working, it may be a pointer to a different sort of distress that needs a different sort of approach. It seemed that the time spent in silent companionship had enabled sufficient trust to develop that enabled him to identify and share the source of his suffering. The re-connection with his son meant that Albert had died healed.

Dr Colin J. Hartree MB BChir MRCGP FRCP
Consultant in Palliative Medicine
St Wilfrid's Hospice, Grosvenor Road, Chichester, West Sussex, UK PO19 8FP
colin@hartree.org.uk

Joyce Holland

AFGOS

When I was in my 50s I attended a new age church where a Nun addressed us. She started with the words "Life is full of AFGOS."

As we pondered on these words she continued "Another Fucking Growth Opportunity."

The phraseology was shocking – but the impact significant.

I began to review my life and realize that I have been "fortunate" to have encountered many AFGOS.

One of the first was when my precious daughter was born. After thinking that I might be sterile after a perforated appendicitis, I gave birth to a perfect baby girl, Jane, after 36 hours hard labor. Over the next 24 hours it was discovered that she had congenital dislocation of her hip and she was placed in a frog plaster for the first 6 weeks of her life. This was my first great lesson in acceptance of life's imperfections. Instead of showing off my perfect daughter to everyone, I had to carry her on my hip and cover her lower half with blankets to conceal the cast.

Life has continued to throw AFGOS to me until my age of 74 and I can honestly say that I appreciate the lessons that they have taught me and believe that they have helped me to be a better and more understanding Palliative Care Physician.

Joyce Holland, MD, Palliative Care Physician
South Fraser Health Authority and Delta Hospice
4407 River Road W., Delta, B.C V4K1R9 CANADA
joyce@jaisbote.f9.co.uk

Andrea Holtzer

What It Means to 'Be There'

In the spring of 2004, my brother-in-law, David, was dying of cancer. He and my sister married three years earlier. This was David's second marriage. They were the proud parents of a beautiful little girl and life held much promise. To say David did not want to die is an understatement.

I was changing jobs and had one week off. There was a long list of things I was hoping to accomplish with this 'free time,' but instead I was called to help with David's care, 200 miles away. At this point I was an RN for 24 years. I was OK with being around and helping dying people. I was ready to talk to David about dying - loss, love laughter - but he was NOT. What he focused on was cure, even though the doctors said this was not possible. There was no laughter, no tears, no heartfelt conversations. Just minute to minute, hour to hour tweaking of medicines, emptying of the catheter bag, managing the I.V.

I was a skilled nurse! I was present when my grandmother died and when my father died. Surely I could help! No way! He wouldn't let me or anyone else in.

I literally went to the library and found books by Dr. Kubler-Ross. She wrote about patients who never found acceptance or found it just hours before death. WOW! I could now deal with this - it was no longer my job to help David accept his terminal illness. This was an enormous relief.

The next problem was a practical one. Although I tried to teach my sister the mechanics of his care, she was **unable** to learn. She is an artist, not a "scientist." I was starting a new job – but do I abandon my own sister and brother-in-law in their hour of need?

Well, I reached out to my dearest friend, colleague and mentor – Win!! She had been a nurse about 40 years and is one of the kindest, wisest persons I know. She helped to put things in perspective. No amount of time was going to change my sister's paralysis. She was dealing with the impending death of her husband – the father of their 35-month old daughter. The sadness permeated every aspect of life, despite our best efforts to provide some sense of normalcy for my niece. We needed a "Plan B."

Win helped me understand that we needed to consider a skilled nursing facility. She urged me to find a place close enough for frequent visits. The burden of caregiving would become the responsibility of the staff and my sister's job would be wife, mother, love, and friend. Another "WOW" moment! We didn't have to do this ourselves. Did my 12 years of experience in home care blind me to other options?

This conversation with my sister went better than I could have imagined. You could see the relief on her face. We had Plan B and it looked OK.

David died in that facility about three weeks later with his family surrounding him. I'm not sure that he ever did accept his terminal illness but this was no longer important. David died in his own way, scripting his own agenda. Did I want more for him? For my sister? You bet. But it wasn't meant to be. And things were still OK.

I've 'been there' for many patients and their families since David's death. I've come to believe that I learn more from the patients and families that challenge my idea of a good death. "Whose death is it anyway" takes on new meaning for me. Believing that options are available and not being afraid to explore them is critical. Thank you, David, for teaching me so much.

Holtzer, Andrea, BSN, RNC
St. Mary's Hospital, Palliative Care Program
17 Minaville Street, Amsterdam, NY, 12010 USA
andreaholtzer@paxway.com

Elizabeth LaRocque

Hospice-Palliative Care IS the Weaned Child on the Lap

[Note to reader – On September 13, 2006 at a community college, Dawson College in Montreal Canada, a lone gunman (Kimveer Gill) went into the school and killed at least one student (Anastasia De Sousa) and seriously wounded at 9 others. The following story is based on these events.]

Recently in church the homilist said he had taught the policeman who *held the body of Anastasia [De Sousa] in his arms.* This brought to mind the powerful image of Michelangelo's *Pieta* statue, the image of a mother holding her dead son on her lap. Apparently the sculptor, in order to depict a full grown human person on another's lap....had to depict Mary like a 250-pound football player: huge.

It does take a Huge-Spirited person to run full of fear, yet fearlessly, into dangerous places where death may come at any second. It sounds like many of those police persons and many students and teachers had this Huge Spirit of supporting and sustaining the lives [and possible deaths] of many at Dawson College recently.

It reminds me of the Davidic Psalm/Song Prayer #131:4 *Like a weaned child on its mother's lap, so* ***is*** *my soul.*

A cousin of mine teaches at Dawson. She and many others manifested this Huge Spirit as she held close to her the lives of several mentally challenged students, forgetting any danger to herself, until they were able to manage on their own. Like weaned children on a lap.

I reach out my hand and place it on the shoulder of that policeman, of my cousin, of the mothers, fathers, siblings, relatives, friends of Anastasia and Kimveer and all the loving caregivers who hold the dying and dead in the lap of their compassion, love and grief. I invite all to stretch out our hands with palms down as a gesture of blessing, of solidarity, of compassion, as we unite with our Jewish sisters and brothers in these holy days of atonement, prayer, and restoration of the Huge Inclusive Spirit of being one on the planet.

A few weeks ago the Montreal and Quebec community, among many others, held the Dawson College community on its Huge Lap.

This past week at Montreal's *Palais du Congres Conference on Care of the Terminally Ill*, 1,500 participants from 38 countries reached out and touched the shoulders of one another as thousands of stories of death, dying, and grief were shared. How many weaned persons per year does the worldwide Hospice Palliative Care community hold on its planetary lap? The numbers grow.

May we all have this Huge Spirit of Mother Earth with weaned children on her lap. May we all have this Huge Spirit of *Pieta*, of Compassion, of Acceptance.

May all beings be one.

Elizabeth LaRocque

End-of-Life Spiritual Care Planner

8343A Blvd LaSalle, LaSalle, QC H8T 1Y6 CANADA

514.365.8275, monkbags4aids@hotmail.com

Suzanne Leece

Joanna's Story

In 1992 I attended the International Congress on the Care of the Terminally Ill for the first time. I had been interested in palliative care for about 8 years and had been looking for opportunities to learn more. This conference was a life-altering experience for me. I have only missed on of these conferences in the years since 1992.

This "success story" occurred just a few months after returning from this very important event. Joanna was in her late 50s. She was a single mother of 9 children, ranging in age from their late teens to early 30s. Joanna had advanced metastatic breast cancer. She weighed about 80 pounds. Her body was showing all the signs of preparing to die. She had not been able to eat for about 2 weeks, had very little urine output, her respirations were irregular, her hands and feet discoloured and cool to touch. She was not able to talk. Yet Joanna could not seem to let go and seemed to be fighting her death.

After observing Joanna and her children for a couple of days, I began to see a pattern. As her children surrounded her bed, there were times when one or two of them would be visibly and audibly upset. As one of her children would sniffle or sob, Joanna's facial expression would change and she would take a deep breath. I began to wonder if what was happening was that Joanna was hanging on because her children were not ready to let her go.

This concept was new to me, having been introduced to it at the conference. I now understood that persons die on two levels: that of the physical and that of the psychosocial and spiritual. Joanna's body was shutting down, but she did not seem ready to leave her body. I had learned that often persons need permission to die and a way of saying goodbye. Was that what was happening here?

I continued to watch this family and began to observe that Joanna's oldest son, Henry, was beginning to show some leadership of his brothers and sisters. I took Henry aside and spoke with him for a few minutes about my observations and the possibility that his mother may need to know that he and his siblings were going to be OK – that they understood what was happening and introduced the thought that she may need them to say goodbye and give her permission to die.

Henry, as the oldest male in the family, turned out to be a "take charge" kind of guy. He immediately gathered his brothers and sisters together and had a talk with them. Each of Joanna's children then spent some time with her, saying their goodbyes. Henry spoke with his mother last. A few minutes later his mother died very peacefully.

I truly believe that it is important to assist family members to understand what is going on as someone is dying. With this knowledge, coaching and support, family members are empowered to do what they need to do – in their own way. When this occurs, often their loved one may die more peacefully.

Working with Joanna and her family thought me the importance of educating and empowering families. My intervention only took a few minutes but I believe that it made a difference in how this family was able to deal with their mother's death and in their own bereavement.

Suzanne Leece, RN, BScN, CHPCN(C)
Certified Hospice Palliative Care Nurse
105 Ontario Street, Brantford, ON N3S 7J7 CANADA
519.759.5010, sleece@bfree.on.ca

Colleen MacDonald

Warm Hands

I wanted to share with you one of the most special moments I have experienced in caring for dying patients. It is not dramatic, or spectacular, but for me a palliative care nurse working in a small town Ontario Hospital, it has had a special place in my heart.

Sara, a seventy-something married woman with two successful grown daughters first came to our unit in the summer, for symptom management related to chemotherapy for breast cancer. She had been battling cancer for six months and her last dose of chemo really took a lot out of her.

Sara was a charismatic woman, active in the community and had many friends. She was kind and quick-witted, always ready to share a laugh. At the time of admission, Sara was nauseated and weak, but uplifted at the fact that the chemotherapy had been quite effective in shrinking the now open tumor consuming her right breast. Unfortunately, she was too ill to undergo any more chemo, so she was referred to a larger center to consult a radiation oncologist. She underwent five doses of radiation as an inpatient at the larger hospital and was then transferred back to the unit where I work.

With every dressing change, we watched in amazement as the tumor continued to shrink. Sara, her family, and the entire palliative team were uplifted by the positive effects the radiation had had. Sara began eating more, building strength and overcoming symptoms. Her pain decreased and her attitude soared. She was beating her cancer! She returned home for, and had another, consultation with her oncologist, who decided to resume chemotherapy as an outpatient. Sara would visit our unit when in the hospital for her chemo. She was always very appreciative of our care and her enthusiasm and joy brought hope and strength for many of our staff. Although I love my job within palliative care, and I find it extremely rewarding to be successful in guiding patients toward a comfortable and peaceful death or controlling patients' symptoms effectively, I found it refreshing to have a patient who's health improved so dramatically.

Sara finished another round of chemo and was able to stay home for another ten months or so, before she returned to our unit. She was very ill, confused and dehydrated. It was next to impossible to get an IV started or blood drawn. She was having more pain and the tumor had begun to grow again since her therapy had stopped.

As you can well imagine, many of the team members were quite upset by this, as it was obvious to us that she was dying. Her family continued to be very attentive and were open to discussions about the fact that Sara life was coming to an end. I am not sure exactly what it was about the situation that pulled at my heartstrings so much. Whether it was the fact that I had a close relationship with this patient and her family, built over time, or that I liked an respected her so much, or that to me she represented hope and strength in the face of uncertainty.

As a palliative care nurse, I have become fairly skilled at assessing patients as they near death and communicating with families so that they can be present with their loved ones if they wish to do so. However, on the evening before Sara died, I would not have guessed that she would only have a few hours to live. Her daughter had spent the night, but was sleeping in the family room at the end of the hall. For whatever reason around three o'clock she woke up and went into the room. After a few minutes I followed her in and we sat at the bottom of the bed and she told me of all the wonderful memories she had of her mother.

Sara's respirations were easy and she was comfortable. We had a quite CD playing in the background with water and birds singing along with classical music. As her daughter shared her precious memories and we giggled together over funny stories, Sara's eyes opened wide and she looked down towards us. We both moved up the bed flanking Sara on each side, each holding her cool hands. She continued to look ahead but was very peaceful and serene, her breathing easy. Her daughter began to pray out loud, and as she did Sara's hands became very warm and I could feel a heat all around her. She took only a few more breaths and very beautifully closed her eyes and died. Her daughter and I spent some time sitting quietly, shared some tears and even some laughter. The heat that I felt when Sara was dying stayed with me throughout the shift and I felt very honored to have shared in such a beautiful and intimate moment in such an extraordinary moment in Sara's life.

Colleen MacDonald RN BScN
Palliative Care Unit, Northumberland Hills Hospital
1000 DePalma Drive, Cobourg Ontario K9A 5W6 CANADA
905.372.6811 x 3219, cmacdonald@nhh.ca

Marie Macková

Guardian Angel

I am a hospice social worker in the Czech republic. I have worked in palliative care for 10 years. I have had many clients during for this time and I have many stories. One is particularly special for me. It is from when I first started in this field.

One month before Christmas I met a woman in the hospice who had breast cancer. She looked very poor and everybody thought that she would die soon. She was 49. I spent a lot of time with her because she did not have any family; only her old parents.

She was an English teacher. Time continued on and she was still alive. She taught hospice staff English. We read books about ethics, philosophy etc. together. Every Friday we had a discussion club in her room.

I built a friendship with her and we became like sisters. More and more we discussed faith and life after death.

One day she asked me, if I would be able to stay with her in her moment of death. I said, "Yes." She asked me, too, if I was afraid of ghosts. I said "No, I am afraid only of being a bad person."

She said, "O.K., when I die I will come back to tell you if there is life after death.

Time continued on and she was still alive. One day I had to tell her that I was going for three months to Britain. She said, "Never mind, I will be waiting for you."

And she did wait. I called her every day and when I came back I called her to say that I was back. That same day, I got a call from the hospice. She was dying. I went over immediately. I was sitting with her and was holding her hand. She died early morning with a smile on her face. She had died 15 months after coming to the hospice.

I went home after her death and my mum told me, "She died and she died at 3.42 a.m." I was surprised because it was exactly the time of her death. My mum sat down and just said, "I was in my bed and I felt somebody sit down beside me. I opened my eyes and I saw a little women. She said, "Thank you" and put her palm on my face. I am sure it was her. I believed it too and I believe she is in heaven. But I feel at the same time, that she is with me if I need help and she is my guardian angel.

Marie Macková PhD., RSW
Hrabenov 115
789 63 Ruda nad Moravou, Czech Republic
Mobile phone: +420 775 224 962, mackova@quick.cz

Balfour Mount

Ten Commandments of Healing

How important to attend to the insights of our teachers, that is to say, the men, women and children who have been our patients and their families. We are indebted to them for the legacy they leave us. Paradoxically, their end-of-life lessons have not been about dying, but about living. What is the core lesson they have taught us? It is that healing is the central goal of life. I am not speaking of physical healing, a person can die healed: what I mean by 'healing' is a shift in our quality of life away ***from*** anguish and suffering**,** ***toward*** an experience of integrity, wholeness and inner peace. Jon Kabat-Zinn defines healing as a process of adaptation, a "coming to terms with things as they are."

The psyche, it would seem, has an intrinsic tendency toward healing, a will-to-wholeness, as it were. How can we experience that? How can you and I find inner peace in the turmoil of each day? Let me summarize our patients' message to us as **"**The 10 Commandments of Healing.**"** They are:

1. Be Truly Present to this Moment

Healing, like love, celebration, awe, wonder and ecstasy, happens in ***the now***, in the present moment, free from ruminations of the past and fears about the future. As Oliver Wendell Holmes stated it, "What lies behind us and what lies before us are tiny matters compared to what lies within us."

And yet I find that I spend most of my time preoccupied with the past or the future. I must come into the present; be aware of the persons and things that are around me ***right now***.

2. Trust

Healing involves letting go, a leap of faith, 'dving not drowning' as Carl Jung expressed it. Lou Gherig's disease patient Phil Simmons called it 'learning to fall.' We fall ***from*** head, ***to*** heart; ***from*** egoism and our carefully constructed defense mechanisms, we fall ***into*** forgiveness of ourselves and others, the realization of the staggering potential of our essential selves, and an awareness of healing connections.

We may experience these connections at four levels: a sense of connection to self (Carl Jung's individuation); connection to others (Martin Buber's 'I-thou' relating); connection to the world perceived through our senses (as with music, or the grandeur of nature); and connection to ultimate meaning, however perceived by that person: God, the Other, the Cosmos, the More, the unity of all things.

3. Attend to Your Whole Person Needs

According to the time-honored metaphoric classification, we are 'body, mind, and spirit', or, 'body, spirit and soul', depending on you preference. We must care for our needs in ***each*** of these domains ***every*** day.

4. Open to Deeper Relating

Recall that our inner life is relational in its expression. It is reflected in how we relate at the four levels noted above.

Within your religious or wisdom tradition seek out teachers who speak from personal experience, not dogma. Go to depth. As C.S. Lewis observed, "The process of living seems to consist in coming to realize truths so ancient and simple that, if stated, they sound like barren platitudes." Lewis continues, "They cannot sound otherwise to those who have not had the relevant experience: that is why there is no real teaching of such truths possible and every generation starts from scratch."

5. Listen to Your Intuition

As Joseph Campbell put it, "Follow your bliss."

6. Create

Identify things you like to do. Make time for your creative side each day.

7. Develop Self-Reflective Skills

Monitor self, noting your thoughts and feelings. They are ***not*** reality. They are your ***response to*** reality. Let go of them and come back to your centre of calm. Work on becoming self-aware with questioning that asks, "What is my personality type and how does that influence how I feel about myself, how I relate to others and to the situations I find myself in? What are my defenses - the walls I build to protect myself, but that also imprison me?"

8. Be Gentle with Yourself

Progression toward healing is slow. Indeed, the goal is never reached. The journey is everything. You are a unique experiment in creation, with a particular potential to contribute to this world. What is it that you alone can do, ***must*** do, if you are to fully express your potential?

9. Think Small

Give up illusions of control. Recognize that we are all in the same boat, ***exactly*** the same boat. The ego-driven values of Western culture ('I am number one'; the need for wealth, power and control; the distrust of all but the physical; the need to be the best in the world in what you do) stand in the way of healing.

Avoid power; neutralize the fantasies it creates in situations where it is bestowed on you. Humility and openness are essential antecedents to healing; joy, peace and a sense of connectedness its products.

10. Celebrate

In the direst of circumstances, boundless peace is to be found within. Recall Viktor Frankl's hard-won observation, "Everything can be taken from a man but one thing: the last of human freedoms – to choose one's attitude in any given set of circumstances, to choose one's own way." If Frankl can find life worth celebrating in Auschwitz, chances are I can find my cup half full, perhaps full to overflowing, here and now.

These are the 10 commandments of healing that our teachers have given us.

* * *

Healing involves a process of opening, slowing, centering, trusting, hoping and accepting. It involves recognizing the potential that still remains, in spite of all that has been lost.

For each of us the path toward healing will be different. The most certain path I have found is meditation. I do not imply that it is the only path. It is just the only path I know. The purpose of meditation, in its many forms, is to create alert awareness with a still mind and presence to the moment.

There is no shortcut to healing. Carl Jung put it this way, "The attainment of wholeness requires one to stake one's whole being. Nothing less will do; there can be no easier conditions, no substitutes, no compromises."

How do we find healing? We must take up the journey anew each day. What better day to recommit than today? No one else can do it for me. No one else can do it for you. Hillel expressed it succinctly, "If I don't do it, who will do it? If I don't do it right now, when will I do it?"

I wish each of you well on your journey.

Mount, Balfour. (September 2006). "Ten Commandments of Healing" in *Selected Journals of Successful Hospice Palliative Care from the 16th International Congress on Care of the Terminally Ill, September 26-29, 2006 in Montreal, Canada*. Toronto: Legacies Inc. with permission from Lawrence Erlbaum Associates. "10 Commandments of Healing," in *Journal of Cancer Education* 2006, vol.21 #1, pp. 50-51.

Balfour M. Mount
Emeritus Professor of Palliative Medicine
McGill University,Programs in Whole Person Care
546 Pine Avenue West, Montreal, Quebec H2W 1S6 CANADA
514-398-2298, wpc.oncology@mcgill.ca

Mary Murray

A Job Where Everybody Dies

I am a hospice home-care nurse in northern New Jersey, about 15 miles west of New York City. Our area is a cultural melting pot. My work has brought me into the homes of immigrants from all over the world.

As part of my caseload, I was the primary nurse for hospice patients in a sprawling complex of brick apartment towers housing mostly elderly Russians who emigrated to the U.S. in the early '90s. Most of these people were older when they arrived in the States, and because the buildings were a nearly self-contained community, they spoke little English. They also held fast to Russian culture, and to beliefs about health, wellness and trust (or lack of) in the American medical system.

One fall day, we admitted to our hospice program a 96-year-old man from the Ukraine. Mr S. was oxygen-dependent and in the last stages of emphysema, but he expressed a fierce desire to maintain his independence as long as he was able. He walked around his apartment with mile-long oxygen tubing and accepted only a few hours a day of help from a health aide.

In Kiev, he had run a factory. Now years later, in Newark, NJ, it was clear he was a man still used to being in charge.

Through his interpreter, a younger man from Azerbaijan working as an aide, Mr. S. told the hospice team how he survived the brutal Battle of Stalingrad, and showed off his World War II medals. He told us about the day he met Khrushchev, and illustrated this story by pretending to bang his shoe on the table as the Russian leader once did at the United Nations.

When a new medication was needed, Mr. S. would patiently listen as the aide translated my instructions. He looked up every new med in his Russian-language drug book. When I would return, a shrug, another polite smile, and most often, no med in sight ... "I no need."

But Mr. S. welcomed visits from the hospice team, and was especially gracious to his nurse. When I would try out a few phrases in my fractured Russian, he would beam and gently correct me ... then encourage me to try again.

The hospice team looked forward to our visits with Mr. S, who inspired us with his stories and dignity. When his 97th birthday drew near, we wanted to celebrate. After we spoke to his aide who got the go-ahead from Mr. S, we decided on a cake and a time for the hospice team to bring him a party. His two nurses and the social worker would attend.

His birthday, Saint Patrick's Day, was cold and rainy. The rain turned the snow on the ground to a dirty deep slush. I wanted to stay in bed. But instead, I slogged out to work, my first stop to buy the cake for our party later.

At my first scheduled visit that morning, I arrived to find the patient near death. I had just a few minutes to spend with the family, gathered around the bed, before the patient took a last, quiet breath. It was obvious the family didn't realize their husband and father had just died. It fell to me to tell them.

Only minutes passed before my pager went off, and I was sent to another home where another person had just died. I knew this family well; the patient was the second in this family I had cared for in the last year.

I had made many visits to this home, and had been helped by the nephew of my patient (himself battling cancer) who had insisted on helping me change a tire when I came out of their house a few weeks before to discover that I had a flat.

When I left their house after Auntie's death on this cold gray day, a party was the last place I wanted to be. But my colleagues were waiting for me in their cars outside of Mr. S's apartment house, and I was late.

We gathered up our cake, paper plates and lemonade and piled into the elevator. I grumbled about the weather. I wondered out loud, and not very nicely to my colleagues, why anybody would want to have such a sad job where all the patients die.

We got to Mr. S's door. I went into nurse mode and knocked.

The home health aide opened the door, smiling and waving us inside like a game-show host. At his usual spot at his little table was Mr. S – no bathrobe today, in a full blue suit and tie. The table was covered with lace. There were Russian pastries and an unopened bottle of wine. The china cups and glassware usually collecting dust on a shelf were washed and sparkling.

At the center of the table was a bouquet in a vase, coffee and three wrapped gifts.

"Come in, my friends," said Mr. S. It was evident he had practiced a speech. "Please, sit down. Happy Birthday to me."

To our social worker (a man), he presented a wrapped gift; a bottle. To my nurse colleague and me, boxes of Russian chocolate. And to me, the flowers from the table. None of us had the heart to tell him we weren't allowed to accept gifts. We thanked him.

"Thank you, my friends. You good for me," he said.

He extended his hand, and I when I offered him mine, he kissed it.

About three months later, on a summer Sunday, Mr. S. died suddenly and without pain, sitting at the same table spooning sugar into a cup of tea.

In that moment when we stepped into Mr S's apartment for that very special party, and whenever since I think of him, I remember (or perhaps that was the day I really learned) why it is that I keep coming to work to do a job where everybody dies.

Mary Murray RN, CHPN
Saint Barnabas Hospice and Palliative Care Center
95 Old Short Hills Road, West Orange, NJ 07052 USA
973.322.4843, maryfmurray@comcast.net

Elizabeth Paddon

Leaving with a Grace

My father left this world with a grace he rarely exhibited when living. Oh, I'm not talking about lying in the hospital for days on end with all manner of tubes sticking out of his body. That was not graceful. Nor am I talking about the awkward dance that we family members made around him as we clumsily tried to make peace with the fact that he was dying. Lots of love there – but no grace.

Grace did come, however, in the ebb and flow of his last breaths. After the doctor turned the ventilator off. After those that did not want to be present had left the room. And after a hushed recitation of the Lord's Prayer and a sweetly sung "Amazing Grace" 'cause he enjoyed that song and it didn't seem quite appropriate to sing his true favorite song "O, how they danced on the night they were wed".

Eternity touched each soul present and guided us to be still. My father's breath became like the waves of the ocean – sometimes calm, sometimes wild – never steady. A soft inhale followed by an exhale so quiet it seemed not really there. *Eternity opens her arms.* A deep inhale followed by a crashing wave. A long silence. A quick breath in followed by a violent exhale. Silence again. I begin to weep. A warmth in my heart reminds me that *I am standing in the presence of Eternity now* – another inhale – this one deep – deep – deep – *Eternity yawns wide* – the body that belongs to my father shudders – *Go to the light, Dad, go to the light* - we say as our hands grip more tightly – and then, a movement so beautiful that only nature could choreograph it. The hands that belong to my father, the hands of the workman, the poet, the angry man and the healer – his hands pull his arms up into a fetal position, and then with the last crashing wave of breath exhaling he pushes down, down, down – as if pushing himself out of his body – pushing, pushing, pushing – until...*it's as if I see him soaring out of his body, shaking his head, opening his arms wide and saying...jeez, it's good to be out of there. That was a hard one. That was a hard life.* I know Dad. But just look at you now. I couldn't stop smiling.

Elizabeth Paddon
Speaker/Storyteller/Singer
Director - Creative Voiceworks
Toronto, ON CANADA
416.593.5009, info@creativevoiceworks.ca, www.creativevoiceworks.ca

Nick Ruiter

A Hospice Client Encounter

I met a man this summer, in his 80s, with a head full of curly white hair.

I sat on his couch with him. I knew his pain was not well controlled because the initial referral from homecare stressed that his goal was "to get the worry out of my system" rather than deal with his physical pain.

I asked him if he was experiencing pain. He grimaced and replied, "I wouldn't wish this pain on my worst enemy." Then he added, "Time's no good for you when you're sick" and he managed a smile.

Such living wisdom is not easy to come by. He has since died but he will be one of my teachers for a long time.

Nick Ruiter
Spiritual Care Coordinator, The Dorothy Ley Hospice
170 Sherway Drive Suite 3, Etobicoke, Ontario M9C 1A6 CANADA
416.626.0116, spiritualcare@dlhospice.org

Mona Rutenberg

Handcasting: Holding onto a Legacy

A few years ago, I decided to combine my knowledge of a casting and molding technique with my work as an art therapist on a palliative care unit in an acute care hospital in Montreal. I had to adapt a technical process, usually done in my sculpture studio, to be easily carried out at a patient's bedside.

I began to present casting a patient's, and at times, a family member's hands as part of an individual's work in art therapy. Basically, by the end of the process, I would be giving the individual or family member a realistic plaster copy of the hand gesture.

For some people, when initially offered the opportunity to leave this type of legacy, they cried but were deeply moved to know that when their loved one is gone, they will be able to retain this powerful keepsake. For others, they have taken the offer as a chance to leave a lasting gift of themselves – a quiet, powerful gesture. In some cases, just watching or participating in the process gives them a chance to be creative, discover something new, and to celebrate life.

Once, while two people had their hands clasped in the rubbery substance, one said when asked to pull their hands out of the mold, "but I don't want to let go." How symbolic of their relationship. It's not easy to say good-bye. But this process helps to deal with the inevitable parting and begin to deal with their grief.

We are familiar with the significance of photographs and how they stir memories within us, yet a sculpture can be held, touched and admired from many sides. The duplication of the hand, in this process, is startlingly real, and for some reminds them of the comfort and pleasure of having once touched and held that hand. The hand that was squeezed, tickled, stroked, clasped and belonged to someone who was cherished.

It is an honor to be part of someone's final days, where perhaps I have helped to ease the pain of saying good-bye. Casting something is not a new technique, but bringing the approach into a hospital and blending empathy, a lending ear, compassion for a fellow soul, respect for the patient and family as they wade in deep waters, gives me satisfaction both personally and professionally.

Mona Rutenberg
5411 West Broadway, Montreal, Quebec H4V 2A3 CANADA
514.481.8314, monarutenberg@yahoo.ca

Mary Anne Schleinich

Reconnecting to Her Whole

When I met Mrs. Dubyk, she was sitting up on her bed, cross-legged, and watching T.V. She had been hospitalized because of pain which had caused her to become largely bedridden for the past two months. Her increasing care needs were a concern to her daughter who lived with her and who also worked full-time outside the home.

I do not recall the medical details of Mrs. Dubyk but I was impressed by the flexibility, strength and energy she demonstrated by sitting in her position. I was also impressed by the great posture she held for an elderly woman and her attention to the cooking program. She did not make eye contact with me, and so I asked her about cooking and our conversation continued with her eyes fixed on the T.V.

I asked her if there were some special dishes she typically made for Easter, a holiday that was coming up. She said yes, and that she was very good at making doughnuts of her heritage. I suggested that an idea might be to make these on the unit. I asked what was needed, and wondered if her daughter might bring in the materials and ingredients.

With some surprise at the request, her daughter brought in the electric frying pan and ingredients later that week. Mrs. Dubyk joined us in the Family Room. She stood and made doughnuts at the table with enthusiasm. Her daughter exclaimed that I was getting her to do something she had never done before, which was to learn how to make these doughnuts from her mother.

The timing could not have been better. Mrs. Dubyk belonged to a group of women from her country of origin, with whom she had both danced and sang for many years. Several of these women came on the unit to visit and entered the Family Room. At once Mrs. Dubyk was connected to the many roles she occupied before her illness. She was mother, hostess, cook, and member of her women's group, linked to ancestral roots.

The opportunity for supervised activity and the Family Room as provided by the Tertiary Palliative Care Unit enabled Mrs. Dubyk to see that her roles endured her illness.

It is possible that grief at loosing her roles contributed to her pain and suffering, and that reconnecting to her whole self-facilitated pain control. She returned home soon afterwards.

Mary Anne Schleinich, BScOT
Occupational Therapist, Tertiary Palliative Care Unit 43
Grey Nuns Community Hospital
Edmonton, AB T6L 5X8 CANADA
780.735.7693, maryanneshcleinich@cha.ab.ca

Ian R. Smith

Ruth: An Interfaith Encounter

A major part of my outreach ministry in the wider community is my involvement as Pastoral Coordinator (volunteer) of the hospice in my area. I have experienced many moments of grace in this hospice ministry, but the following story is perhaps one of my most memorable to date. Any names used are fictitious to protect the identity of the persons involved.

* * *

"Ruth", in her mid-to-late 70s, was a patient in the hospice for about four months (a much-longer than usual stay than most of our patients). She was Jewish.

The first day I met her, I introduced myself as the Pastoral Coordinator of the hospice, and that I was also a full time Christian pastor. I subsequently saw her once or twice a week until about a week before her death. We talked about all sorts of things, and she was very open to sharing her spiritual journey.

During our second or third encounter, Ruth smiled and said to me, "I hope you understand that, while I accept that Jesus was a good man - perhaps even a prophet - I cannot accept him as my messiah."

I responded, "I'm not here to convert you, Ruth, I'm just here to share God's presence with you." Over the next few weeks, we had some incredible faith talks.

About a week before she died, I went into her room and she looked deeply troubled. I said, "Ruth, what's on your mind today?"

"Death," she responded in a flat monotone.

"Would you like to talk about it?" I asked. And so we did. She was greatly troubled about having to leave her loved ones behind.

And then, suddenly, she interrupted herself and said, "Will you pray for me?" ... and so, holding onto her hand, I began to pray, thanking God for the support of her loved ones around her; for all those things in her life that had reflected God's love; and that God would ease her pain at having to let go. I then began to sing a gentle Hebrew blessing in English ... "May the blessing of the Lord be upon you...".

Her eyes were closed, and suddenly, her hand began to shake in mine. Her family members in attendance gathered around the bed, thinking she was about to die. With her eyes still closed, Ruth looked up and began shaking her head back and forth, saying, "No, not yet! ... not yet!"

After about three minutes of this, she opened her eyes and gave me a puzzled look. I asked, "Ruth, did something just happen?"

"Yes! I saw light and what looked like blurry human shapes, and they were wanting me to go with them, and I told them I wasn't ready to go."

"How did you feel when you experienced this?" I asked.

"I wasn't afraid; it was very peaceful ... beautiful really," she responded, "but I wasn't ready to go with them."

Ruth died about a week later ... about an hour before I happened to enter the hospice for the Weekly Rounds meeting. The family was waiting for the funeral home to come and pick up Ruth's body.

One of her daughters came up to me and said, "It was amazing! My mom was comatose, and I was lying beside her in the bed, holding onto her. Dad was standing at the foot of the bed, and my sister and brother were sitting in chairs right next to the bed. Suddenly, Mom woke up with an incredible glow on her face ... looked at me and smiled ... then smiled at my sister and brother ... then smiled at my Dad ... and then looked up over Dad's head ... uttered an exclamation of wonderment and said 'Uncle Mike!' ... and breathed her last. It was so beautiful!"

("Uncle Mike" was Ruth's beloved uncle from Europe where she grew up. He had died about 40 years previously. Both of her grandfathers had died when she was little, so Uncle Mike had taken on the role of her grandfather).

* * *

Some conventional, traditional interpretations of Christianity would say that the possibility of such an occurrence is out of the question ... because Ruth was not a Christian. What has been reaffirmed for me from this spiritual journey is that, being open to encountering Ruth as she was, being open to being an instrument of God's presence, and being open to wherever that might lead, I ended up on very "holy ground" ... an experience I will cherish and celebrate for the rest of my life. Our patients are, indeed, our best teachers.

Rev. Ian R. Smith
30 Saddlewood Avenue, Pointe-Claire, Québec H9R 5S6 CANADA
514.626.4795, ian.iansm@gmail.com

Janet Stark

Coming Home

Dad was dying. He was a retired farmer from Southern Ontario and he was dying of lung disease.

One spring day we got *the call*. It was my Mom, asking us to come to Hamilton to the hospital. Dad had gone on oxygen a few days before at home, and now his condition was worsening. At one point his heart had stopped, and with a flurry of activity he was revived. At the time, the doctor didn't know he had a hand-written advanced directive with a *do not resuscitate* order.

In retrospect, my Mom said it was just as well, as giving him a few more days of life allowed us to say our good-byes.

All five children made it home, and at one time all of us were in the hospital room with Dad. We're spread out now, and it's not often we are all together. Dad knew he was dying. I had written him a poem, thanking him for all of the things he taught me over the years.

Garnet Law 1925-2005

Dad
Over the years you taught me many things
To play euchre, checkers and crokinole
To dance, and enjoy fiddle music
To make homemade ice cream
To like black licorice and humbugs
How to braid binder twine for a calf rope
To swing on a rope in the barn
How to write a speech about Wilf Carter

To sing to the cows: "Mares Eat Oats," "Little Brown Jug,"
"Turkey in the Straw" and "Cheer Boys Cheer"
To enjoy a country picnic
How to feed a dog from the table
A strong work ethic; (I picked stones)
To take interest in my family history
To take pride in the love of the land.
For all these things I am grateful.
I love you Dad,
Janet

He was not an emotionally-expressive man, but as I read him the poem that night, he squeezed my hand so hard. Without words, I knew he loved me, and he had given me the blessing. He said *thank you* and it was more than enough.

One afternoon, we all went down to get a snack and give Dad some quiet time. When we returned, his minister was there. The minister had my poem in his hand. They must have been chatting about us kids, because I heard my Dad say *I guess we didn't do too bad, because all his kids came home to see him.* The minister was doing what we call in palliative care: *giving meaning and purpose by a life review.*

Over the next few days, there were lots of family going in and out of that room, and at one point we thought he had rallied and was improving. When the doctors discussed palliative care with my parents, it was then that Dad said he wanted to go home. The weekend was coming, and it was going to be hard to arrange his discharge with home nursing care. It was month end as well, and the doctors were on monthly rotation. He was getting a new doctor too. We promised him we would get him home.

He held on, weak with very labored breathing and not able to eat much. Late Tuesday afternoon, the ambulance brought him home. As the attendants carried the stretcher into the old stone home, he had them stop and he took a long last look at his farm. He looked at the fields and the rolling hills, the barn and the home where he had brought my Mom as a new bride fifty-five years before. Again he said *thank you*. They put him into the hospital bed, which had been prepared in the living room. Then it quieted down.

My Mom was with him, and also my sister, a geriatric nurse. Perfect. His breathing changed, and with my Mom and my sister holding his hands, he died, about an hour and a half after he got home. It was *perfect*. He had come home, to his beloved farm, to die.

Janet Stark CHA
Lanark, Leeds & Grenville Palliative Care Education Coordinator
Brockville General Hospital
Garden St. Site, 42 Garden St. Brockville ON K6V 2C3 CANADA
613.345.5645 x 4414, staja@bgh-on.ca

Anna Towers

Touch Their Hand Gently

I have a useful clinical tip for palliative care professionals! This is something that our Palliative Care Head Nurse, Rhoda Hoffman, taught me back in 1993 at the Royal Victoria Hospital in Montreal.

Often when we make our rounds on hospital or inpatient hospice patients, they are, or seem to be, asleep. We never wake patients up, but what if they're not really sleeping?

What a dilemma! Rhoda taught me to touch their hand gently. If they open their eyes, they weren't asleep, only resting. And if they're deeply asleep, a light touch on the hand will not wake them. Dilemma resolved, nobody gets awakened from precious sleep!

Dr. Anna Towers
Director, Palliative Care Division
McGill Departments of Oncology and Medicine
1650 Cedar Ave, L10.221.3, Montreal, Canada H3G 1A4 CANADA
514.934.1934 ext 43964, anna.towers@muhc.mcgill.ca

Harry van Bommel

Let's Go for a Walk

"Let's go for a walk" has started many of my conversations with family members, friends and colleagues who want to talk about their worries, questions, and feelings about the dying process. I have found that a walk (or a drive when a walk is not possible) is one of the safest ways to talk about some of our most difficult feelings and thoughts.

It is safe because we can talk without looking directly at each other. It is safe because we can walk for minutes without having to say a word. It is safe because when we want to cry, we can put on arm around each other's shoulders, stop and hug if we like, or just keep walking -whichever is most supportive.

I remember walking with a friend whose mother was dying. We were walking along downtown streets in mid-afternoon with all the hustle and bustle that implies. Yet we were walking in almost complete isolation. We did not really see much of what was happening around us. We felt alone in a crowd and it felt comforting somehow.

Walking in no particular direction with no particular goal in mind, we talked about some general feelings, thoughts and observations on the weather, the news reports of that day, etc. The conversation slowly, and naturally, moved to where she talked about how much she worried about her mother's care, her concerns about possible pain and discomforting symptoms, and her worries of how the rest of her family would deal with her mother's death.

We took each of her concerns in turn and I gave her some ideas of what might help in each situation and we brainstormed other ideas. We discussed which local hospice program might meet her mother's needs best and how to establish a support circle of family, friends and neighbors should her condition continue on for some months. We discussed effective pain and symptom control and what barriers might exist in her mother's situation that would need to be addressed. She talked, at length, about her family dynamics and with only a few opened-ended questions on my part, she examined what was possible to achieve in the weeks that remained and what was likely not to be resolved within her family.

When we walked by an art gallery, she interrupted our conversation to tell me how her mother used to take her to galleries and museums to share her passion for the arts and history with her. She talked about her parents' lives together, their accomplishments, their difficulties and how they overcame some of them, and their love of family. There were many memories of love as well as some of disappointment. There were memories of not meeting her mother's expectations and others of moments together sharing a cup of tea or discussing a common book they were reading. Tears were often in her eyes. It was clear that her mother meant a great deal to my friend and that she would dearly miss her.

We walked in silence at various times without any sense of pressure for either one of us to talk. Silence, amid the noises of the city, was possible and necessary and comforting.

We talked about how she might fill some of her time with mother in ways that would be especially meaningful to both of them. We talked about what she might do with her mother now to provide her wonderful memories in years to come – memories that would provide strength, comfort and even joy when my friend might need them most. Things as simple as reviewing photo albums together, writing a poem or letters to each other, listening to music quietly while snuggling up by the fire. Holding hands. Sharing a tissue box. Telling stories.

Not altogether conscious of how our walk had turned into a circular route, we were near her home where we had started. The last half-hour or so we had walked a lot in silence. She had said most of what she needed to say and asked the questions she thought I might have answers that could be helpful to her and her family. We enjoyed each other's quiet company along the tree-lined streets in her neighbourhood – each deep within our own thoughts. She about her situation – me thinking back to times with my mother and father before they died.

In her driveway, we hugged, cried a bit at all the experiences she had gone through in the past months and the ones yet to come. She smiled and said a thanks and I smiled and thanked her as well. These types of walks are a mutual gift of trust, of sharing practical information and of listening with the heart and mind and spirit. We both offered insights and thoughts that are helpful to the other. We both accepted the help and consolation that the other offered unconditionally.

Dr. Dorothy Ley said that at the heart of successful hospice care is spiritual care. In her words, "It says we are here. We will be with you in your living and your dying. We will free you from pain and give you the freedom to find your own meaning in your own life – your way. We will comfort you and those you love – not always with words, often with a touch or a glance. We will bring you hope – not for tomorrow but for this day. We will not leave you. We will watch with you. We will be there."

One practical way of doing this is to say to someone "Let's go for a walk." If they can no longer walk, perhaps a drive will work. If they prefer or need to stay at home in a chair or in bed, then simply sit kitty corner to them. Be close enough to touch them when appropriate yet not directly across from them so they can look away from your eyes easily and with no guilt when they need the "space" to be alone for a few minutes with you right next to them. This is one of the true joys of hospice palliative care and I feel blessed each time I can share in such a memorable conversation. A gift of hospice palliative care is the time we give ourselves to be with people in silence, in conversation, in harmony.

Harry van Bommel
Executive Director, Legacies Inc.
11 Miniot Circle, Toronto, ON M1K 2K1 CANADA
416.264.4665, *harry@legacies.ca*

Index

Adams, Lucie 11
art 57
being there 33
brother-in-law relationships 33
Chaban, Michéle 15
chemotherapy 40
children 25, 38
community 21, 25, 36
cooking 59
Corbier, Melanie 21
Cottle, Margaret 25
Dawson College shootings 36
father-daughter relationships 54, 64
Fillmore, Cathleen 27
grace 54
handcasting 57
Hartee, Colin 30
healing 45
Holland, Joyce 32
holocaust survivor 15
Holtzer, Andrea 33
immigrant 50
interfaith experiences 56, 61
LaRocque, Elizabeth 36
last moments of life 38, 54
Leece, Suzanne 38
lessons learned from new circumstances 32, 45
letting go 38
lonely 50, 56
MacDonald, Colleen 40
mother-daughter relationships 21, 27, 40
Mount, Balfour 45
murder 36
Murray, Mary 50
opportunities 32
Paddon, Elizabeth 54
pain 30, 56
poetry 64
prayer 61
radiology 40
roles, valued 59
Ruiter, Nick 56
Rutenberg, Mona 57
Schleinich, Mary Anne 59
singing 15
Sisters 11, 33
Smith, Ian R. 61
spirituality 43, 61
Stark, Janet 64
suffering 30
time, our short times with people 11
Not helpful 56
touch 67
Towers, Anna 67
van Bommel, Harry 68
waiting to die 43
walking, as a communication skill 68
wisdom 45, 56

The Essential Hospice & Home Care Library

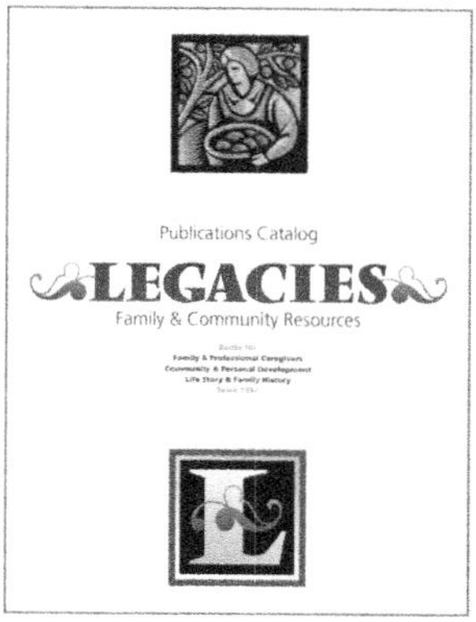

For a complete list of Legacies books,
request your catalog today!
http://www.legacies.ca

.....

Selected Journals on Grieving

King's College 16th International Conference on Death and Bereavement
Edited by Harry van Bommel

Professional and volunteer grief therapists share their personal and professional stories about grief and bereavement during this 3-day conference at King's College, London, Ontario. The stories can be used in your own practice, newsletters and presentations as illustrations of how others deal with their grief.

Leo Tolstoy wrote that every time we write we should leave a bit of our blood in the ink pot. The stories in this book do exactly that. The stories are thoughtful, personal and a great testament to the importance of human relationships in all their many forms.

The stories in this book look at: views by professionals about their work; personal stories by spouses, parents, children and siblings; spiritual aspects of care;

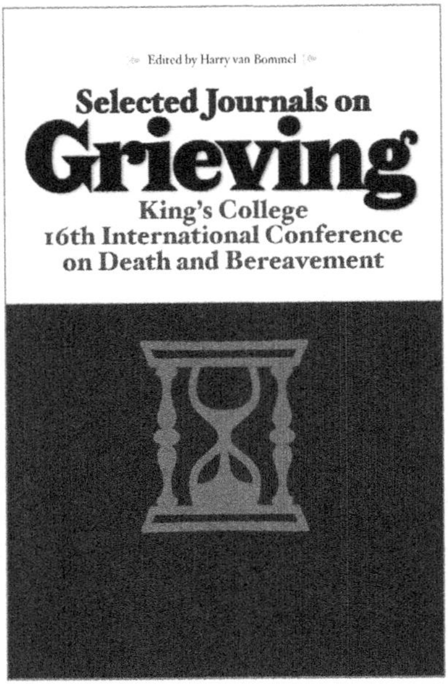

the importance of animals in people's lives; philosophical musings; and so much more.

Each story is a short vignette of a person's journey through grief. These are stories about practical things that people have done to help others or to help themselves. One or more of these stories will touch your heart because we have all grieved the death of someone we love. In reading how others have dealt with such loss, we identify how we are coping and what we need to continue to do to help others while also looking at things we might want to do differently so that we don't hurt ourselves or others we love.

This material was gathered at King's College 16th International Conference on Death and Bereavement in London, Ontario, Canada. Everyone who has participated in the project has ensured that their stories are free of error and respect the confidentiality of the people involved as necessary. They retain copyright for their own stories and accept responsibility for what is recorded.

84 pages, 6 x 9 inches, ISBN 1-55307-024-0, $20 paperback, $15 ebook

. . . . .

The Heart of Hospice

Dorothy Ley with Harry van Bommel

The spiritual heart of hospice as well as other aspects of the hospice philosophy of care are cronicled. Includes a biographical sketch of Dr. Dorothy Ley, a Canadian and international pioneer of the hospice care movement, with photographs.

"Spiritual care lies at the heart of hospice. It says we are here. We will be with you in your living and your dying. We will free you from pain and give you the freedom to find your own meaning in your own life - your way. We will comfort you and those you love – not always with words, often with a touch or a glance. We will bring you hope - not for tomorrow but for this day. We will not leave you. We will watch with you. We will be there." - Dorothy Ley

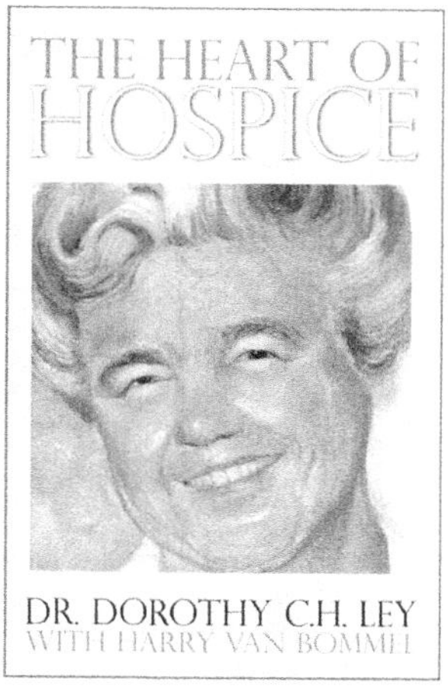

The Heart of Hospice provides a useful and inspirational educational tool for palliative care providers primarily but also for everyone interested in palliative care. The insights of one of the pioneers in Canada are practical, direct, humorous, colorful and inspirational. Her experiences lend a practicality and a credibility to this work that is hard to find elsewhere. Best of all, we can learn from someone who actually practiced what she taught. She was a very human role model to physicians, other health care providers, family members and now to patients.

The book is divided into three parts. The first part includes the Introduction and the two chapters on the pillars of care and Dr. Ley's personal comments to people within palliative care. Her words are a compilation of various speeches and articles that she wrote over the years about the importance of providing physical, emotional, spiritual, and information supports to people with a life-threatening or terminal illness and their families. They are her words supplemented by information collected during conversations with Harry van Bommel. The second part describes some hospice care success stories including the excellent hospice care that Dr. Ley received in her own last months of life. The third part is a collection of information that readers may find helpful in understanding both Dorothy Ley and her message.

The book is called The Heart of Hospice because Dr. Ley understood the often forgotten spiritual element to palliative care. In a real sense, her belief in, and promotion of, palliative care and her experiences as a doctor, family member and patient put her at the heart of hospice as well - a well deserved place in the history of this young movement.

135 pages, 5-1/2 x 8-1/2 inches, ISBN 1-55307-022-4,
$20 paperback, $15 ebook

About Legacies

Legacies: Family and Community Resources was founded as a not-for-profit Canadian corporation in 1999. It's mission is to support individuals, families and communities in creating meaningful legacies through community development, hospice and home care, and Canada 150, our project to encourage Canadians to record their life stories and family histories. Harry van Bommel and Janet Klees are the founders and directors.

Legacies has a simple philosophy:

1. Stay small and think big.
2. Use volunteers whenever possible and, when necessary, collaborate with thoughtful, committed and determined people.
3. Reach the widest audience possible with information that is practical and immediately useful.
4. Recognize and encourage the mutual exchange of people's gifts for the betterment of individuals, families and communities.

Legacies: Family and Community Resources
11 Miniot Circle, Scarborough Ontario M1K 2K1 Canada
Telephone 416.264.4665 Fax: 800.684.7280

Legacies is on the web at: http://www.legacies.ca

Made in the USA
Monee, IL
04 November 2026

67378981R00046